WHY AM I SO TIRED?

WHY AM I SO TIRED?

TRISTAN EVERGREEN

CONTENTS

CHAPTER 1

Introduction to Fatigue

Fatigue is one of the most common complaints people express. It can be mild and infrequent or it can be severe and occur frequently. It can result in dysfunction. Fatigue can be a very significant and sometimes permanent disabling symptom. Fatigue, in general, refers to a subjective, often very distressing state of feeling tired or exhausted—more or less than usual because of either too much mental or physical work. When people complain of fatigue, they are usually not referring to short-term tiredness, but to a lack of energy and ache, lethargy, and diminished ability to perform necessary tasks. Understanding and managing the discomfort of unusual fatigue can be complicated by its many causes, which not only can be physical but can also be psychological and psychosomatic.

Busy life and societal demands require all of us to juggle many jobs and obligations at once—often inviting a work-life imbalance by not eating right, not sleeping enough, and not exercising enough. Juggling seems impossible and more often leads to feeling heavy, tired, confused, and with no appetite for most enjoyable events. These are some of the symptoms that may manifest as surprisingly vacant physical and mental energy that are collectively known as fatigue. Furthermore, hearing a complaint of fatigue in a friend or coworker invites reactions based on mood and perception of the urgency of the day (e.g., "me too," "trying to keep up with the rat race," "part of getting older," etc.). It can also be hard to understand or be supportive unless you have experienced chronic fatigue yourself.

Defining Fatigue

Fatigue is a common condition that most people will experience at various times. It is a complex phenomenon with many contributing factors, including being physically exhausted, having sore and tired muscles, and experiencing mental and psychic strain. Fatigue is not the same as sleepiness or even tiredness, although an excess of any of these conditions will compromise psychological functioning and wellbeing. Fatigue refers to the subjective feeling of exhaustion and is viewed as having both physical and mental components. It is also a conditioned feeling, in that some physical exertion is required to trigger the alert. Practically speaking, fatigue can manifest as a reluctance to initiate physical activity, a shortened endurance for physical activity, or, in the worst cases, an inability to continue with physical activities.

Our understanding of excessive fatigue is still in its infancy. However, for this subbenchmark, excessive fatigue is understood, and it can arise from three main physical states or a combination of them. Firstly, hypercapnia, the presence of carbon dioxide in the body occurs. Secondly, hypoxia, the lack of oxygen usually because of ischemia, can occur. Thirdly, hypoglycemia, a lack of glucose, can impair brain function, although the science is yet to explain this phenomenon fully. Effects of fatigue describe the human reaction to increased feelings of tiredness, including the associated effects on cognitive and sensory processing, decision-making, and psychological and physiological functioning. Furthermore, the effects of fatigue are viewed as a continuum of increasing severity from reduced efficiency through to impairment and dysfunction.

Types of Fatigue

There are several different types of fatigue, each with unique causes and implications. Acute, temporary fatigue is the normal byproduct of exertion, whether physical or mental, and is expected in healthy individuals. It is relieved through proper rest and recovery, and its long-term effects can be mitigated by equal attention to self-care and stress reduction. Chronic fatigue refers to a more sustained period where energy resources are depleted, occurring for over six months despite rest and sometimes due to prolonged physical or emotional tension. Chronic fatigue may also be a symptom of underlying medical or psychiatric conditions, including cardiovascular or respiratory disorders, autoimmune issues, cancer, obesity, diabetes, anemia, infectious diseases, endocrine disorders, sleep disorders, alcohol and substance abuse, nutritional deficiencies, and mental health concerns.

Chronic Fatigue Syndrome (CFS) is a potentially distressing type of tension-induced chronic fatigue where no underlying physical or psychiatric condition has been identified. It has complex and varied symptoms, but primary symptoms may include persistent fatigue, memory problems, reduced mental processing speed, sore throat, unrefreshing sleep, tender lymph nodes, muscle or joint aches, and significant post-exertional malaise (lasting longer than one day but not meet criteria for CFS). Sometimes, what feels like fatigue is not fatigue at all. Boredom or burnout is a possible outcome of disengagement and shallow thinking within an unstimulating work or home environment. Depersonalization or dissociation with basic tasks may produce feelings of "feeling like a zombie." Certain energy lifescapes or energy "crashes" can be caused by chronic self-imposed restriction or prohibitively low food intake, leading to feelings that "my muscles are heavy."

CHAPTER 2

Causes of Fatigue

Fatigue can consume a person's life and make it hard to overcome the simplest of tasks. The physiological makings of this symptom are complicated, for they result in neurobiological, psychological, social, and physical factors. Physically, the body experiences fatigue as a result of specific deterring factors. It accumulates damage to both muscle and connective tissues, reduces one's pain threshold, and creates metabolic and thermal strain via a variety of biochemical and thermoregulatory processes. Psychologically, it can be perceived through a combination of neuronal activity, conscious thoughts, motivation, and behavioral aspects. Correlating the causes below to the individual can help a person understand their own condition in more depth. Despite individual experiences, we are all subjected to the same general instigators.

Physical causes of fatigue range from the classic tiredness after exercising to tiredness from doing labored mental work, working a demanding job, reduced blood flow, pain, inactivity, amount of body fat, poor diet, or others. There are many psychological factors that may contribute to fatigue. Chronic anxiety and hyperarousal put the body into states of constant vigilance, and one spends their time agonizing over the "what ifs." Depression and fatigue are inextricably linked. Depression is sometimes masked by fatigue, making it harder to diagnose. Depression reduces one to a shell of their former self and affects the way one perceives, feels, and experiences life to crisis proportions. It creates altered beliefs, thinking, and a bombardment of negative thoughts. Experience with oneself has proven further traits of fatigue symptomatology, including sex role, masculine and feminine qualities, body image, sleep attitudes, other personality traits, and social capital.

Physical Causes

Looking at a person's life and taking note of a few things they are involved in or have to deal with, fatigue seems to come as no surprise. From the multiple engagements, they reluctantly find themselves in to the worrying events that keep them awake at night, the question seems not to be if they deserve to be tired, but more of how they should be tired. What exactly is the source of this widespread weariness?

Physiological Underpinnings of Fatigue. Among the factors that have been highlighted in a confluence of studies to predict fatigue, illness (chronic or transient, especially infections) has been found to be the most consistent determinant. This is unsurprising, considering that the psychological sensation of fatigue is only its experiential expression and occurs due to disturbances in the body, particularly in the brain. It has been shown that indicators of oxidative stress in the blood and upregulation of inflammatory biomarkers in the body, which can result from free radicals and reactive oxygen species being formed under disease conditions or during exercise, are associated with fatigue. Moreover, endocrinological pathways in the brain, which control the actions of virtually all cognitive and behavioural targets, can be affected by inflammation during increased brain activation, leading to a feeling of tiredness. Thus, it follows that in situations of increased oxidative damage, such as during physical disease or exercise, a partition of the necessary resources in the brain to have them dedicated to inflammation, defence, and repair (jointly called sickness syndrome) will result in fatigue or, at least, attenuation of motivation. In some cases, the motivation to respond to certain physiological needs regarding homeostasis can become enhanced (thirst, salt craving, etc.) as has been shown to occur with short-term exercise.

Psychological Causes

Fatigue and tiredness are complex, multifaceted experiences. Psychological aspects play a significant role, the most blatant example being stress-related physical exhaustion. When we are completely drained on a psychological level, we also feel the fatigue physically. In psychology, the classic distinction is made between emotional, cognitive, and naturally, motivational elements that are said to produce the human experience of fatigue. These causes are often mutually dependent – emotional downers are often automatically accompanied by cognitive dissuasion and sometimes even produce bodily symptoms. If we want to understand why we often feel so tired mentally, we need to shed light on this complex interaction.

One big block negating mental energy is the cognitive rumination that can occur when troubling thoughts churn round the same issues without getting anywhere. Researchers have found that rumination spots some issues and thinks about them continuously. They are often unsolvable in principle, which naturally frustrates the muser further. Additional physical exhaustion combines with the existing psychological exhaustion resulting from these ruminatory adventures. It is thought that pondering the negatives in life is not conducive psychologically. It seems particularly likely to provoke feelings of helplessness, exhaustion, and despair. Of course, too much of any specific cognitive strain will produce fatigue. The classic opponents to fatigue are the cognitive stimuli that we consider modifications of the executors that teem with energy: We feel secure mentally and so can get absolutely everything done. There are also people with extremely high standards who are exhausted by overseeing far too much, winding themselves up into the state of a perfectionist burnout.

CHAPTER 3

Impact of Fatigue

Fatigue - phenomenally common in the modern world - has the ability to alter both our brain and our body, placing us at greater risk of diseases ranging from colds and flu to obesity, diabetes, and cardiovascular disease. Over and above the physical and biological effects of fatigue, being tired frequently simply makes life less enjoyable. The categorization of sleepiness as a disorder, and the realization that the standard treatment - chronic use of stimulants - is not truly effective in terms of protecting against accidents, has driven medical researchers to determine what states of being tired are doing to bodies and brains.

The implications of this work extend far beyond the clinic. All sorts of life circumstances and conditions can bring on the same profound weariness. At work, employees can be fatigued not only by their efforts but by their lack of efforts. The FOMO effect of constantly monitoring phones is well-documented, producing the real-world consequence of people sending more and more emails that say less and less. With so many people low in mental resources, and rational self-interest so dominant, is it any wonder that we are finding it harder to put ourselves in someone else's shoes? Current human resource management initiatives of promoting 'engagement' miss the methodological potential of tiredness: if the adults are tired, they might lack the relevant mental resources to understand your customer complaint, or to design a study that reliably finds out which of your policies really works. Moreover, while motivation as engagement might be easily dismissed as the 'myth of worker passion', manager policies of 'promoting well-being' while restructuring a workplace may inadvertently be suggesting that fatigue is a personal weakness when, given the circumstances, they are an entirely rational response. In addition to distancing insights from folk dualism, a genuine scientific advance would bring us far closer to Marx's socialist dream of "...a society in which the full and free development of every individual forms the ruling principle". With real science, our policies and practices can start from where we all are, not where we politically wish that we were.

On Physical Health

Fatigue can have pronounced effects on functioning and quality of life, increasing the likelihood of workplace accidents, car crashes, difficulties in school, and functional impairments among healthy individuals as well as those with chronic disease. Fatigue can also interfere with mental functioning, leading to impairments in cognitive and executive functioning, and a variety of emotional disturbances. Understanding the physical impacts of fatigue is critical to devising appropriate interventions, particularly when the general purpose of such interventions centers on maintaining or improving physical health.

Intervention programs focusing on lifestyle components such as physical activity or nutrition often target conditions such as obesity, cardiovascular disease, diabetes, and other chronic illnesses that are known to be related to various types of fatigue. In addition, some standard approaches to chronic disease management include learning to manage energy and manage symptoms on a day-to-day basis, which can significantly impact both mental and physical fatigue. For example, doing daily checklists to conserve energy, starting with making the bed in the morning versus gathering dishes after dinner or reorganizing your closet at any time of day, and blocking out periods of time for quiet rest can all help manage fatigue at a number of different levels. Similarly, nonpharmacological interventions that help individuals relax, such as deep breathing, yoga or meditation, can reduce symptoms of depression, improve focus, and reduce discomforts associated with fatigue.

On Mental Health

The mental health side effects of prolonged fatigue and tiredness cannot be understated. Overwhelming exhaustion can significantly decrease your capacity to resist and stave off negative emotions, and leave you feeling emotionally raw. Because fatigue can make it hard to find the motivation to get out of bed, let alone participate in activities that you enjoy, it can increase feelings of low mood. Likewise, relentless fatigue can disrupt your concentration, attention, and memory processes, leading to doubts about your capability and levels of anxiety.

Guilt often sits atop the hearts of people wrestling with exhaustion. You may feel remorse for succumbing to fatigue, or for needing to share the burden with others. The pandemic, with its accompanying stress and grief, has served as a perfect storm for the generation of masses, fueling feelings of fatigue and mental ill-health. Now more than ever, it's crucial to approach and research fatigue in holistic ways, not just scientifically but also in terms of its implications for an individual's mental health and their broader quality of life. To do justice to "tiredness," we need to focus on people's subjective experience of low energy, questioning how they suffer and where this suffering comes from. It's through this that we can begin to understand the humanity at the heart of the "cry" of tiredness.

CHAPTER 4

Assessment and Diagnosis of Fatigue

The assessment and diagnosis of fatigue are of immense importance. First, accurate identification is crucial to address the consequences of fatigue. Second, individualized management of fatigue in cancer patients is impossible without an assessment and diagnosis. Yet exploring fatigue is labor-intensive because the issue is complex.

The assessment of fatigue generally entails quantitative and qualitative measurements that provide a detailed insight into the scope and nature of patients' fatigue. In developing the psycho-oncological guideline to treat cancer patients, Kuhnt et al. (2014) proposed a systematic procedure for evaluating fatigue. The guideline caucus proposed using a decision algorithm for detecting physical, emotional, and mental fatigue in cancer patients, and suggested the procedure might also be fruitful for detecting and diagnosing fatigue stemming from causes other than a cancerous development.

An overview of the proposed algorithm. First and foremost, anamnesis is essential. It allows for clarifying and delimiting the duration, beginning, and variances in fatigue as well as promoting an understanding of relevant constellations. Clarity is required with respect to the distinction between fatigue and exhaustion, for example. Physical, mental, and emotional factors may underlie fatigue experiences. Interestingly, mental fatigue is not generally associated with sleep disorders, though it might be associated with insomnia.

The approachability, applicability, practicability, acceptability, implementation, and sustainability of the proposed algorithm would have to be tested in clinical practice to prove its viability as a reliable procedure. Moreover, the decision-making steps in the proposed algorithm are based on expert ratings and consensus that has not been empirically tested.

Medical Tests

To address fatigue, your doctor may order specific tests to measure hormone balances, vitamin and cholesterol levels, and thyroid function; liver and kidney function; and the big ticket—certain infectious diseases. People with diabetes can display those signs and symptoms as the result of their disease and may need their treatment changed, although they may also have the syndrome. A sleep study could be warranted if you have excessive snoring, leg movements, or episodes of gasping for breath during sleep that awaken you during the night. A tilt table test, which can help determine if you have POTS, starts with lying on a table while you are hooked up to an electrocardiogram (ECG), a monitor that measures electrical activity of the heart. Then the table tilts to about 60 to 80 degrees while your doctor and nurses monitor you for signs of fainting.

Doctors conducting this test can give you medication to block the effects of certain receptors in the body, reducing the chance of fainting, and they might also use nitroglycerin, a chemical that lowers blood pressure, to aggravate symptoms if they're suspected to be present and hiding just below the surface. An echocardiogram can provide further information about heart function. People with unexplained fatigue often ask for tests to evaluate for subclinical, as well as overt, autoimmune disorders. Major organizations and physicians who take care of individuals with autoimmune diseases do not recommend this testing in the absence of signs or symptoms consistent with an autoimmune disease. Brain MRIs aren't typically recommended unless you have neurological deficits, such as weak muscles, problems with speech or memory, or are at high risk of developing neurological issues based on your history or genetics.

Questionnaires

Questionnaires can be used to assess a patient's fatigue, which can be helpful in the profiling style of understanding a patient's needs. They may encompass what some authors have called "fatigue severity" i.e. how bad is the fatigue including some cognition components and they also capture the patient's interpretation of this lack of energy and inclusion of activity-related factors. Self-reporting of fatigue can provide an overall view of a person's interpretation of their fatigue and can add invaluable insights into how they manage on a day-to-day basis including: work, household tasks and taking part in leisure activities. This is a complex area and the questionnaire tools that are available to us at the current time are also complex and can be multi-faceted. The weakness of a questionnaire with such depth in qualitative analysis is the amount of work required to interpret these findings within a clinical area that is time sensitive.

Patients with M.E./CFS (Myalgic Encephalomyelitis/Chronic Fatigue Syndrome), for example, often have severe fatigue. By using a combination of questionnaires and healthcare professionals, we can begin to build up an understanding of the patient's entire fatigue experience, from descriptive features to influencing factors. When we add to this the experience of a pain consultant the data becomes clinically relevant, patient-specific and will include areas that a patient mentioned that may not be discussed with another patient as the individual's fatigue experience is so diverse.

CHAPTER 5

Treatment and Management Strategies

Given the diverse range of factors that can contribute to fatigue, it follows that the treatment and management for fatigue should follow a corresponding, multi-faced approach. Not only do individuals suffering from fatigue need to identify which of the various factors are responsible for their symptoms, but they will likely need to combine and use a range of different strategies to effectively manage their symptoms.

1. Lifestyle Adjustments This might result in needing to reduce hours in work, change to a less physically or mentally demanding role, or ceasing work entirely. It could also involve making adjustments to our living situation to reduce the number of things we need to do in our daily lives. For example, by introducing a cleaner or gardener, or living with family members who can pick up some of the slack. Although this strategy can lower stress and prevent further fatigue, it is unlikely to be able to raise energy levels when someone is currently experiencing symptoms of fatigue.

2. Dietary Strategies It is less clear how much of a role dietary strategies play in fatigue that does not involve exercise. In addition, the small changes seen from the studies attempting to manipulate di-

etary factors may be the results of low to moderate quality studies, meaning we are not entirely sure if the effects on fatigue are due to the dietary factors that have been altered. Over the next several years, we should learn more about dietary strategies for symptoms of fatigue through CFS/ME research.

3. Physical Activity and Exercise

4. Sleep Optimization

Lifestyle Changes

Almost as if you're hearing words tap-dancing along your delicate brain matter, lifestyle changes are an integral aspect of managing fatigue. The unexpected truth about a Rubenesque dose of daily exercise is that it's your best hope for recovering lost energy. Exercise can help increase your energy levels, focus, and overall capacity for activity over time while also increasing the probability that it releases endorphins into your doughy, cashed-out muscles and helps reduce your pain and risk of developing depression. It's best if your exercise is tailored to your specific physical health, daily schedule, and preferences. Like a sloth avoiding predators, take your time easing into new routines and back off when you need a bit of rest. Sitting all day while drafting an epitaph of your wasted vitality? Make it a priority to get up and move around every thirty minutes or so, even if it's just to engage in some moderate physical theatre. Take the time to figure out what vegetation works best for you, and what it's like! After the plants, try to schedule a nighttime period, preferably one that's about seven to nine hours long, in which you aren't doing zesty dance routines. Light-blocking curtains, earplugs, low light levels, feeds, and cool air may help to boost the julienne of your slumber. Warm baths or soothing liquids can help your body slow down and get ready for sleep, too.

Planning and organizing may ensure that your energy is being transmitted to the most important parts of the day before an exhausted molasses haze sets in. Isolate the important stuff from the less important. Smart assistants, alarms, calendars, and making the most of your doe-eyed larks can help you in this journey. Multitasking may seem more like something a hyena would use to pickle his after-dinner treat, but it feels helpful. Anidulia, or fatigued nesting, generally leads to more weariness and stress. File down those icky expectations, myths, and unnecessary emotions crowding up your brimming brain-in-a-jar. Trying to find time for books upstairs or existential dread stacking up like Mrs. squishy and obtrusive root vegetables? Make some extra time to binge cool foods. Cut down on the stuff you need to do to an almost dangerous amount. Prioritize the duties that are non-negotiable and involve restful activities as well as the things in your out-of-order pile. Say "yare yare daze" to a 100% packed day. By allowing additional time for transitions and time to sink deeper into pleasurable activities, go for an 80 percent approach instead. Predicting your movements in a person with a lengthy blue haze at your side is much like tapestry weaving. Try to anticipate when you will need to be as active and as awake as possible and when less activity is acceptable. You won't be driving around a hamburger factory if you know you feel tired at about half past lunchtime.

Diet and Nutrition
Nutrition plays an essential role in helping reduce accidents, minimize errors, and promote overall health and productivity in arduous work. There are three broad areas of interest: macronutrients, supplements, and specific constituents that may possess properties such as sedative or stimulating action. While at an acute level, there is limited direct evidence, the suggestion is that a diet high in fiber, vegetables, fruit, carbohydrates (e.g., oats, brown rice) with adequate

high-quality protein, moderate to low in fat, and balanced across the macronutrient energy fields is likely to help maximize vitality. Key minerals with respect to muscle and brain function and energy production include magnesium and iron, both involved in oxygen transport, and iron, in particular, in the production of ATP, a key requirement for energy. Zinc, cortisol, and B vitamins may help prevent any unnecessary increase in cortisol in high-staking virtual reality games, a state associated with stress and hence mental fatigue.

Further, field studies have noted a significant association between regular meals, increased fruit and vegetable consumption, and reduced fatigue in managers. It is just right to find the cure for physical energy and mental vigor in the 'kitchen,' however explained. Dietary habits and patterns appear to have an effect mainly on PCF in food and a small decrease with Deduction, perhaps more likely to keep PFC concentrated. Even minor changes in the daily diet in terms of breakfast food taken influence on life and work, mainly due to the increased interest in breakfast and healthy food. Specifically, it has been observed that the concentration ability of the main oscillated from an average of 31% (in Control breakfast) to 47% and 52% (respectively in Celery breakfast and Carrots breakfast); a 6% (Carrots breakfast) and 21% (Celery breakfast) increase in concentration ability was similarly against control.

Exercise and Physical Activity
The previous section has outlined in detail how chronic physical inactivity can cause extreme fatigue, an insight of potentially immense relevance to fatigue biomarker research, psychophysiological assessments, expert systems, and the development of tailored regimens of physical activity - ones that already have some genuine penetration around the world for implementation in the workplace. At the very least, this section elucidates the importance of exercise for

ameliorating fatigue and preserving, or more accurately, reconstituting energy.

Psychophysiological Effects When an untrained person begins to engage in low-level exercise, the usual negative effects reported are transformations in emotions and physical feelings: these include calm, increased energy, reduced tension and fatigue, and improved mood. When fatigued engines might be expected to sputter and stall, it seems that exercise whips them back into shape. The benefits of low-intensity exercise for those who are otherwise low in mood and fatigued or drowsy have been reported for decades - a boon for those clouded by non-specific fatigue far removed from the elite boundaries of, say, metabolite accumulation. In a wonderful schizophrenic contradiction, effort that starts out fatiguing or increases in fatigue can also have an invigorating effect, a compensation that seems to be partially due to primary personality characteristics: extroverts find exercise more energizing than introverts, for example. Indeed, quite a few studies have reported the same: that fatigue as far-removed as CFS responds well to exercise interventions.

Sleep Hygiene

Having a consistent sleep-wake schedule is crucial for maintaining good sleep hygiene. Go to bed and wake up within an hour of the same time every day. People whose work schedules do not allow for this level of regularity should try to stick with the same bedtime as often as possible.

Address "sleep bullies" in life—be they in the form of light, sound, temperature, a partner, or kids who interfere with your sleep. Even neutral sound—like a distant radio—can hinder sleep, so it is best to use earplugs or a white noise machine (available at many stores that stock electronics), especially if the world is a noisy place or you have family members or roommates whose adventures impede your shuteye.

Keep naps earlier in the day and relatively short—ideally, limit napping to 30 minutes in the morning or in the early afternoon, if you need to nap at all. Do not nap at all in the evening.

Physical activity is essential for healthy sleep. However, it is best to finish exercising at least 3 hours before turning in, especially if you are prone to sleep disruption. Avoid vigorous exercise like running or intense cardio right before bed. Although a post-dinner walk may help digestion and metabolism, it is best to save longer and/or more intense workouts for earlier in the day. Heated exercise, like hot yoga or going for a run when it is hot outside, may make sleep a bit more difficult since thermoregulation plays a role in signaling the body to prepare for sleep.

Many different aspects go into properly taking care of yourself. One of the most important aspects is to develop a habit of good sleep hygiene. Enough hours of sleep, of good quality, at the right times, are the bedrock of a person's proper functioning. Sleep is the body's time for recovery and repair. When we sleep, we heal. This is one of the reasons he believes that sleep is so implicated in savoring.

CHAPTER 6

Coping Mechanisms and Support

As with any chronic condition, there are certain coping mechanisms that let a person manage their fatigue. If you are feeling very tired, at the extreme end of the energy spectrum, read the section, 'What Can I Do Right Now?' for some practical help. However, most of the advice here is for those of you living with a tiredness that may not disappear completely. Support becomes crucial as the effects of fatigue impact on daily life. Paradoxically, giving you this information may be the single best thing you need. Recognizing and understanding your problem is the first and most important step to alleviating the impact on your life. Talking to someone about how tired you feel and what it means to you is also important. We all need a support network of some kind and for some people that means friends or family members.

Some people find support groups useful or talking to others online or over the phone who experience similar things. The organizations listed at the back of the booklet can tell you about support groups, self-help and other resources that may be available in your area. Because of the endless physical, psychological, emotional and situational barriers reducing energy and increasing tiredness, the reader does not only require a better physical functional level that can cope with complete physical and mental exhaustion, but is also in need of coping mechanisms to help distract attention away from their constant battle with fatigue. Therefore, the reader is less consumed by the symptoms of fatigue, making the so-called 'spare capacity' channel more energy to other activities and concerns.

Stress Management Techniques

Because stress is a leading cause of fatigue, it's vital to learn how to manage and adjust your stress coping strategies. The following stress management techniques are not exercises to increase energy, but they can reduce stress and make your fatigue easier to manage. Stressors may not change, but you can change your emotional reactions and coping mechanisms. Some possible ways for you to cope include:

- Psychotherapy: While dealing with fatigue, individuals often feel depression, anger, anxiety, isolation, and loss of control. Psychotherapy interventions may be designed to reduce the emotional impact of persistent tiredness and cultivate a greater sense of vitality. A cognitive-behavioral framework might be particularly helpful, allowing your therapist to guide you in changing mood-behavior patterns that are perpetuating your emotional struggle with fatigue. Within a supportive framework, a therapist can use problem-solving techniques to address barriers to effective stress management and increase your personal coping resources. - Reducing unnecessary stress when possible: Many individuals who feel fatigued try to keep doing the same thing at the same pace they were managing before they began feeling tired. Others may try to get even more done to keep from feeling guilty. For some, this way of coping is a way of proving to others that they are still okay. This stress will only increase your fatigue. Help yourself by identifying the stressors you can control and let go of those you can't.

Support Groups and Counseling

Many people who have chronic fatigue, like ME/CFS or FM, say that only other people with a chronic illness really understand what they're going through. If this is true for you, you may want to seek out a support group for people with chronic illnesses. Either way, a few sessions with a professional counselor can be a big help. They can help you adjust to your illness and guide you in talking to your employer, your family, your friends, and your physician about your fatigue. Many people with chronic fatigue impairments go through stages much like people who have suffered a major loss. The same is true for many people who have chronic pain.

Friends, family, and neighbors generally mean well but are often at a loss as to how to help you. They may even wonder if you're malingering or imagining your fatigue. Despite their good intentions, they may wind up saying things or reacting in ways that hurt you. They may also find it hard to understand why all your dreams and plans have been shattered by fatigue. If your community has a chapter of a self-help organization that deals with chronic fatigue or chronic pain, you may want to consider attending a few sessions before making a decision about whether it's for you. If you do attend, try to keep an open mind about the benefits of group therapy. Look for a group in which members respect one another's need for privacy.

CHAPTER 7

Preventive Measures

General, the following are preventive measures. These measures can apply to many different conditions and individuals with different needs, but the primary goal is to proactively disrupt a pattern of energy-zapping activities. This way, we are preventing any onset of, or setbacks to our low-level symptomatology that is manageable with our treatments.

Rest up. Sufficient sleep is essential for both physical and mental recovery. Sleep improvements can be made from changes to the timing and environment, reducing the intake of stimulants and medications, or stress management strategies.

Diet and Nutrition. Develop an eating schedule to keep your metabolism level, and provide better energy for your day.

Stress Management. Decrease your reactivity to or perception of stress. Consider mindfulness, deep breathing, guided imagery, meditation, listening to music, medication, professional counseling, acupuncture, and biofeedback. Plan time to do something enjoyable or relaxing.

Work Environment. Balance the amount of mental and physical effort expected of you at work. Breaks should occur about every 50 minutes for 10 minutes. Arrange your work environment to be ergonomically accommodative and request accommodation for physical and sensory needs that other coworkers may not have.

Physical Activity. Small manageable portions of physical activity every day help to increase energy levels. Inhibit over-exertion or over-heating you may experience and include active games into your daily routine. Have a range of activity choices to modify to your desires on days when you feel poorly or are managing a schedule that is abnormal for you.

Medications and Other Therapy. Take medications only when necessary and for the prescribed ailment. Use medications appropriate for your symptoms and adjust for age and dosage level, if appropriate. Participate in therapies to control your chronic illnesses (ex: pulmonary rehabilitation or home exercises for chronic lung disease, exercise/weight-lifting program for fibromyalgia). Keep and follow a written plan to track symptoms and commonalities as pertains to fatigue.

Cognitive Behavior Management. Conceptualize a plan to control activity level based on individual symptoms together with a health professional.

Emotional Needs. Address concerns of anger, fear, grief, and depression—any feeling that causes a preoccupation with poor health. Euthymia (happiness) and a serious interest in life are beneficial in the path to living at your best.

Healthy Habits

The only way to defend against ongoing feelings of exhaustion is to actively cultivate habits that promote and restore a sense of physical and emotional well-being. Once symptoms of overload persist, it is likely that the body will continue to signal its stress. Should it go unattended, in the worst cases, this can lead, over time, to conditions like high blood pressure, heart disease, or stroke. These latter are also related to overeating or eating unhealthy foods when comfort is sought or when energy is required to restore mental health; excessively anxious, apathetic, or irritable interpersonal interactions that can wear us down; postural difficulties, upper body pain, weight gain, and sleep disturbances when sedentary for long periods of time; and excessive use of caffeine, nicotine, and alcohol to manage negative feelings. It should be emphasized that healthier choices add up and help us out in times of fatigue. As we get older, experts remind us that the body has its own influence on the way energy ebbs and flows from day to day.

While it may be more difficult for some people to build healthy habits and make a change for a variety of reasons—personal and professional, social and economic—looking after your body, brain, and mental health is an investment that pays off in our capacity to meet life's demands. Therefore, while an early start at an older age is essential, it is not at all impossible. Supplement caregivers' and seniors' perspectives on normal aging and provide information on rebuilding habits to enhance the energy transfer process and reduce fatigue. Training caregivers in the benefits of older adult counseling and coaching approaches, including motivational interview-based techniques and action planning support. Identifying what "healthy eating" and "moderate exercise" mean in practical terms in relation to our daily lives. They also discuss sleep management and its relationship to good sleep and its efficacy. Explaining these habits will not free up more of our days by making them automatic; instead, they discuss them as ways to build up reserves or extra energy to get us through the day when we've had a setback.

Workplace Ergonomics

Office and workplace environments play a large role in the development of fatigue. Incorrect desk and computer screen height, exposure to bright or artificial light, and inhospitable ambient temperatures are all small factors that can add up and contribute to higher perceived fatigue. Workplace ergonomics can address a number of these factors with just a few simple recommendations. This is not a design guide to your new corner office (lucky you), but rather a layman's primer of the humanity-based ergonomics that can make office work really work for you.

The work setting impacts fatigue and fatigue perception. The modern worker can spend up to eight hours a day interacting with their computer workstation. Many workplaces also provide variable start and end times around daylight, artificial lighting may affect fatigue or fatigue perception. Other factors such as office temperature, the presence or absence of drafts, as well as atmospheric conditions (smell and noise) can also have an effect. In industrial physical work settings, the ability to adjust work pace has also been shown to improve fatigue perception and included in most fatigue interventions. Some organizations include these and other factors (such as psychological support and the ability to adjust to a particular level of comfort) when considering the effect of the workplace environment on fatigue. Unfortunately, many other organizations do not, and as a result, many people are exposed to fatigue in the workplace on a regular basis.

CHAPTER 8

Conclusion and Future Directions

The preceding chapters spell out a number of conclusions about fatigue, as well as some proposals and suggestions for ways of preventing and treating it. Although fatigue can be a serious problem for many individuals, it is often not taken seriously - either by the individual herself or by those on whom she depends. One of the most important aspects of this volume is its demonstration that fatigue is real, that it results in significantly altered performance and reduces an individual's quality of life. Nobody should be criticized for being tired; instead, we need to examine the root causes of the fatigue and search for ways to alleviate or prevent it.

The chapters on pathophysiology and clinical approaches to fatigue are clearly meaningful. That is, it is essential that we further the study of fatigue in the hope that an intelligent analysis of the development and structural and functional problems that result from the condition will allow us to prevent or treat it. Although this volume does not provide definitive answers to all of the important questions it raises, it provides an excellent beginning for the quest of understanding how to reduce fatigue in individuals dealing with brain disorder. Considering the complexity and vast scope of the issue, further research is mandatory in order to gain comprehensive understanding. Fatigue is not only a physiological necessity of life; it is also a too frequent outcome of brain illness. Finally, chronic stress can lead to poor mental health, often experienced as symptoms of anxiety, depression, and post-traumatic stress disorder. Treatments for such poor mental health include both psychotherapeutic and pharmacological possibilities. Additionally, an experimental field of research targets novel pharmaco-therapeutics to prevent and fight stress-related disorders.